Hemp Oil CBD (Legal in all 50 United States) vs. Medical Marijuana©

By

Othniel Seiden, MD

A Pachyderm Publishing Publication
All Rights Reserved
© Copyright 2017 by Othniel Seiden, MD

Published in the USA by
Pachyderm Publishing LLC™
Denver, Colorado

No part of this book may be reproduced or transmitted in any form or by any means, electronic or mechanical, including photocopy, recording or by any information storage and retrieval system, without permission, in writing from the publisher.

Find us on Facebook at
www.facebook.com/PachydermPublishingColorado

Also at
www.PachydermPublishing.com

ISBN-13: 978-1975869601

ISBN-10: 1975869605

Cover design by Shosh Seiden

Edited by Rodney Swift

Contents:

1. What Is Hemp Oil CBD, and How Does It Differ From Medical Marijuana?

2. Conditions Benefiting From Hemp or Marijuana

3. History of Cannabis as a Medicine

4. Considering Hemp Oil CBD over Marijuana as Medication

5. Hemp and Marijuana Delivery Methods

6. Who Should Not Use Hemp Oil CBD or Marijuana?

7. Why Marijuana was Made Illegal in the United States

8. Is Cannabis a Gateway Drug, or Addictive?

Look for other books in this Hemp Oil CBD series as they are published. (See Page 113 for details on book titles)

Chapter 1.

What Is Hemp Oil CBD, and How Does It Differ From Medical Marijuana?

What is hemp oil CBD?

Hemp oil CBD is derived from the seeds and stalks of the hemp plant. ***Cannabidiol*** (or ***CBD oil***) is a natural botanical derived from this amazing plant, concentrated so that it is high in the compound CBD.

There are over 85 cannabinoids that have to date been identified in the cannabis plant, and CBD is the second most common after ***tetrahydrocannabinol***, or ***THC***.

However, unlike THC (the mind-altering cannabinoid found in marijuana), CBD is non-psychotropic and does not cause the euphoric high experienced from marijuana use. CBD hemp oil is extracted from the cannabis varieties that are naturally abundant in CBD, and virtually lacking in THC.

The virtual absence of THC in the hemp plant, and in the hemp oil extracted from it, is what allows hemp oil CBD to be **legally used and sold in all 50 United States**. Unlike medical marijuana, in states where it is legal, hemp oil CBD can be purchased without prescription, medical marijuana cards, or any other restriction. Yet, hemp oil CBD has the same medical characteristics, benefits and advantages as medical marijuana. Because it requires no special taxes or licensing to sell it, hemp oil CBD is far less expensive then medical marijuana. In some places it sells for 10% of what medical marijuana would cost for the same derived benefit.

How does hemp oil CBD differ from Medical Marijuana?

Hemp oil CBD is extracted from the ***hemp plant***, a close cousin to the marijuana plant. The marijuana plant contains both CBD (the most active medicinal ingredient in medical marijuana) and THC (the most mind-altering ingredient in marijuana). The hemp plant, on the other hand, contains high levels of CBD identical to the medicinal ingredient of marijuana, but virtually none of the mind altering THC of marijuana. It is this virtual absence of THC which allows hemp oil CBD to be legally saleable and usable in all 50 of the United States, and most of the world.

Benefits of CBD oil

Decades of research indicate that the cannabinoids, like CBD, interact with the body's endocannabinoid system, a complex system that contributes to a variety of biological processes including the body's inflammation responses, relaxation, sleep, appetite, and many other functions. By linking with the two main types of cannabinoid cell receptors, known as **CB1** and **CB2** (found on cells throughout the body), CBD interacts with the endocannabinoid system, helping it in the regulation of the body's natural state of balance.

Like the plant itself, CBD cannabis oil is derived from the hemp plant, and contains only trace amounts of THC. Marijuana, on the other hand, contains and produces a high THC product, causing the user its mind altering high.

Some genetic varieties of hemp contain higher concentrations of

CBD than others. Hemp cannabis varieties naturally possess higher levels of CBD, and these hemp stalks and hemp seeds produce organic hemp oil that is naturally rich in medically active cannabidiol.

Because organic hemp oil is extracted from high-CBD/low-THC cannabis, it doesn't produce psychoactive effects the way THC does, making it a safe and legal option for all age groups.

Medical marijuana and hemp oil CBD are used to treat an enormous number of illnesses and ailments in all age groups, from birth to patients in their 90's and older.

But due to the lack of the THC component in hemp oil CBD, the product is safer in a vast majority of cases.

Chapter 2.

Conditions Benefiting from Hemp or Marijuana

Let's look at some of these diseases and conditions that are benefitted by hemp oil CBD or medical marijuana use:

1. It has long been used in the treatment of glaucoma.

Marijuana has been used successfully to treat and prevent the eye disease *glaucoma*, which causes damaging pressure changes within the eye that can damage the optic nerve, possibly causing loss of vision. According to the National Eye Institute, marijuana is known to decrease the pressure inside the eye. Studies done in the early 1970s showed that marijuana, when smoked, lowered intraocular pressure in people with normal pressure, as well as those with glaucoma. These effects of cannabis have been shown to slow the progression of the disease and prevention of blindness.

Always check with your ophthalmologist when pursuing a new treatment program.

2. Hemp CBD or marijuana may reverse the carcinogenic effects of tobacco and improve lung health.

Hemp CBD or marijuana do not appear to impair lung function if used orally or is vaporized, and can in some instances increase lung capacity, according to a study published in *Journal of the American Medical Association* in January 2012. Researchers, while looking for risk factors of heart disease, tested the lung function of 5,115 young adults over the course of 20 years. Tobacco smokers lost lung function over time; however, pot smokers actually showed a marked increase in lung capacity. It might be that the increased lung capacity was due to taking deep breaths while inhaling the drug, rather than a therapeutic chemical in the cannabis.

3. CBD can control epileptic seizures.

When marijuana or hemp extract (synthetic marijuana) was given to epileptic rats, it rid the rats of the seizures for **up to 10 hours**. Cannabinoids control seizures by binding to the brain cells responsible for controlling excitability and convulsions by regulating relaxation.

These cannabinoid extracts also decreases the symptoms of the severe seizure disorder known as ***Dravet Syndrome***. A five-year-old girl named Charlotte Figi has Dravet Syndrome, for which her parents are giving her marijuana extract to treat her numerous daily seizures. During his research for the CNN documentary *Weed*, Dr. Sanjay Gupta interviewed the Figi family, who treats their 5-year-old daughter using a medical marijuana strain high in cannabidiol CDB and low in THC. Untreated, Charlotte would have numerous daily seizures and severe developmental delays.

Charlotte's treatment has decreased her seizures from 300 a week to just one about every seven days. Now numerous other children in the state of Colorado, where the treatment is legal, are using the same strain of marijuana to treat their seizures. Physicians who recommended this treatment say the cannabidiol interacts with the brain cells to quiet the excessive activity that causes these seizures.

4. Cannabinoids seems to stop cancer from spreading.

*"The CBD in cannabis may keep **cancer** from spreading"* was what researchers at California Pacific Medical Center in San Francisco reported in 2007. *"It seems cannabidiol stops cancer by turning off a gene called **Id-1**"*, was reported

in the study published in the journal *Molecular Cancer*. Cancer cells make more copies of this gene than non-cancerous cells, helping them spread throughout the body. Researchers studied **breast cancer** cells in the lab that had high levels of the Id-1, and treated them with cannabidiol. Following cell cannabidiol treatment, they had decreased Id-1 expression and were less aggressive spreaders.

Further evidence of cannabis's effect on cancer is suggested in Dr. Sanjay Gupta's CNN special *Weed*, mentioning a few studies in the U.S., Spain, and Israel that suggest the compounds in cannabis could even kill cancer cells.

5. Hemp oil CBD and medical marijuana decreases anxiety.

In 2010, researchers at Harvard Medical School suggested that that some of medical marijuana's benefits in pain and nausea relief, the two main reasons it's often used for the side effects of chemotherapy, may actually be partially due to reduced *anxiety*, which smokers note improves their mood and acts as a sedative in low doses. Beware, however, higher doses may increase anxiety and may cause temporary paranoia. The lack of THC in hemp oil CBD tends to avoid this side effect of higher doses.

6. THC slows the progression of Alzheimer's disease.

That marijuana may be able to slow the progression of ***Alzheimer's disease*** is suggested in a study led by Kim Janda of the Scripps Research Institute. This 2006 study was published in the journal *Molecular Pharmaceutics*, and found that THC in marijuana slows the formation of amyloid plaques by blocking the enzyme in the brain that makes the amyloid. These plaques are what kill brain cells, thus causing Alzheimer's disease. The effect of CBD in this study is not clear.

7. The drug eases the pain of multiple sclerosis.

Marijuana has proven to ease the painful symptoms of multiple sclerosis, a study published in the *Canadian Medical Association Journal* suggests.

Jody Corey-Bloom studied 30 multiple sclerosis patients suffering painful contractions in their muscles. These patients' symptoms didn't respond to other standard treatments, but after smoking marijuana for just a few days they were in considerably less pain. The THC in the cannabis binds to the receptor cells in the nerves and muscles to relieve the pain. The chemical also helps control the severe muscle spasms. The role of CBD in this study is not clear.

8. Other types of muscle spasms could be helped too.

Other types of muscle spasms also respond to marijuana. In Sanjay Gupta's CNN report, he found a teenager who was using medical marijuana to treat diaphragm spasms, which were found to be untreatable by all conventional and very strong prescription medications. His condition is called ***myoclonus diaphragmatic flutter***, or ***Van Leeuwenhoek's disease***, which causes non-stop spasms in the abdominal muscles. These spasms are not only painful, but they interfere dangerously with breathing and speaking. Smoking marijuana calms his attacks almost immediately by calming the muscles of his diaphragm. The role of CBD is not clear in this situation.

9. Medical marijuana dramatically eases side effects from treating hepatitis C while increasing treatment effectiveness.

The treatment for **hepatitis C** infection is difficult to endure; its harsh negative side effects include extreme fatigue, severe nausea, intense muscle aches, loss of appetite, and depression. Treatment and its side effects last for months. Patients are often unable to finish their treatment course because of these side effects.

A 2006 study reported in the *European Journal of Gastroenterology and Hepatology* stated that 86% of patients using cannabis successfully completed their Hepatitis C treatments, while only 29% of non-users completed their therapy. Cannabis not only reduced treatment side effects, but also appeared to improve treatment effectiveness. Statistics indicated that 54% of those patients using cannabis in conjunction with therapy got their viral level lower and kept them low, compared to only 8% of non-users.

10. Cannabis can be used to treat inflammatory bowel diseases.

Cannabis appears to benefit ***Crohn's disease***. Crohn's disease is an inflammatory autoimmune bowel disorder that causes pain, vomiting, severe diarrhea, weight loss, and a variety of other symptoms. A recent study in Israel showed that smoking or vaping cannabis significantly reduced Crohn's disease symptoms in 10 out of every 11 patients, and actually caused a complete disease remission in five of those patients. It is admittedly a very small study, but with stunning results. However, other research has shown similar results. The cannabinoids seem to help the bowel to regulate bacteria and intestinal function.

*"Patients with inflammatory bowel diseases like Crohn's disease and **ulcerative colitis** benefit by cannabis use"*, according to research at University of Nottingham found in 2010. The chemicals in cannabis, the THC, and the cannabidiol CBD interact with cells playing an important role in bowel function and immune system responses. This study was published in the *Journal of Pharmacology and Experimental Therapeutics.*

11. Cannabis relieves the discomfort of arthritis.

*"Cannabis relieves pain and reduces inflammation, which helps to relieve pain and discomfort for people with **rheumatoid arthritis**"*, researchers announced in 2011. It also promotes sleep, which arthritis pain tends to interrupt. In a study that further supports this, researchers from rheumatology units at numerous hospitals gave their patients Sativex, a cannabinoid-based pain medicine. After just a two-week period, people on Sativex had a significant reduction in pain and much improved sleep compared to patients on placebos.

12. Cannabis helps your sugar metabolism, and seems to help keep weight down.

A study published in the *American Journal of Medicine* suggested that marijuana smokers are skinnier than the average, and have healthier metabolism of sugars, this in spite of often eating more calories because of the "munchies" cannabis tends to cause.

This study was of more than 4,500 adult Americans, 579 of who were current marijuana smokers, those who had smoked during the past month. About 2,000 had admitted using marijuana in the past, while 2,000 others in the study had never used the drug. The researchers studied their response to eating sugars, their levels of the hormone insulin, and their blood sugar levels while they hadn't eaten in nine hours, and again after eating sugar. Not only were the marijuana users skinnier, but also they had a healthier response to the ingested sugar. The role of CBD in this study was not clear.

13. Cannabis improves the symptoms of lupus.

Medical cannabis is being used to treat the autoimmune disease *systemic lupus erythematosus*, in which the body starts to attack its own tissues and organs for unknown reasons. The chemicals in marijuana seem to have a soothing effect on the immune system, which is probably how it deals with symptoms of lupus. Further positive impact of the cannabis is due to its effects on pain and nausea.

14. Marijuana soothes tremors for people with Parkinson's disease.

Research done in Israel shows that cannabis significantly reduces the pain and tremors of ***Parkinson's disease***, and markedly improves the sleep for patients. Above all, most impressive was the improvement of fine motor skills among the patients.

Medical marijuana is legal in Israel for many conditions, thus a great amount of valuable research into the medical uses of cannabis is done there, and the research is supported by the Israeli government.

15. Hemp CBD and marijuana helps veterans and victims suffering from PTSD.

The Department of Health and Human Services recently signed off on a proposal to allow study of marijuana's potential for treatment for veterans with *post-traumatic stress disorder*.

Marijuana is already approved to treat PTSD in some states. It is interesting that in New Mexico, PTSD is the number one reason for people getting a medical marijuana license. This is the first time the U.S. government has approved a proposal that incorporates smoked or vaporized marijuana, which is still classified by the government as a drug with no accepted medical applications. Israel again leads in research for the use of PTSD having used it for some time in the treatment of holocaust survivors and their own military veterans. Cannabis appears to help regulate the system that causes fear and anxiety in the body and brain. It dramatically reduces recurrent nightmares.

16. Cannabis has been shown to protect the brain following a stroke.

Researchers from the University of Nottingham show that cannabis may help protect the brain from damage caused by *stroke*. Marijuana appears to reduce the size of the area affected by the stroke as shown in rats, mice, and monkeys.

This isn't the only research that has shown the neuro-protective effects of cannabis. Some research shows that the plant may help protect the brain after other traumatic events such as concussions.

There is some evidence that marijuana not only protects the

brain, but also can help heal the brain after a concussion or other traumatic injury. A recent study in the journal *Cerebral Cortex* showed that at least in mice, marijuana lessened the bruising of the brain and helped with healing mechanisms after a traumatic injury.

Of great importance to sports medicine, Harvard professor emeritus of psychiatry and marijuana advocate Lester Grinspoon recently wrote an open letter to NFL Commissioner Roger Goodell, saying that the NFL should stop testing players for marijuana, and instead the league should start funding research into cannabis's ability to protect the brain. "*A growing number of doctors and researchers believe that marijuana has incredibly powerful neuro-protective properties, an understanding based on both laboratory and clinical data,*" he writes. In response, Goodell recently said that he'd consider permitting athletes to use marijuana if medical research shows that it's an effective neuro-protective agent. The role of CBD alone in this is not yet clear.

17. Cannabis can help eliminate nightmares.

For people suffering from **serious and recurrent nightmares**, especially those associated with PTSD, cannabis can be helpful. Nightmares and other dreams occur during **REM** (rapid eye movement) stages of sleep. Cannabis tends to interrupt REM sleep, so those dreams may not occur. Research into using a synthetic cannabinoid showed a significant decrease in the number of nightmares in patients with PTSD. Additionally, cannabis may be a better sleep aid for patients than some other substances people use to promote sleep, such as prescription medication and alcohol.

18. Cannabis reduces pain and nausea from chemo, and stimulates appetite.

One of the most recognized medical uses of cannabis is ***for cancer patients undergoing chemotherapy***. Most cancer patients treated with chemo suffer from painful nausea, vomiting, and loss of appetite, which can cause additional health complications. Marijuana can dramatically reduce these side effects by alleviating pain, decreasing nausea, and stimulating the appetite. An increasing number of oncologists are now actively suggesting cannabis in conjunction with chemotherapy. The role of CBD alone in this is not clear.

19. Cannabis can help people trying to cut back on drinking, and other addictions.

It is somewhat ironic that while some people consider it to be a gateway drug, marijuana is actually used by many **to curb their addictions**. Marijuana is far safer than alcohol; it is much less addictive and doesn't cause nearly as much physical damage to the body and its organs. Research reported in the *Harm Reduction Journal* shows that some people use marijuana as a less harmful substitute for alcohol, prescription drugs, and the illegal drugs.

Among of the most common reasons for patients and addicts to make a substitution to cannabis are the less adverse side effects from marijuana, and the fact that it is less likely to cause withdrawal problems. You might say it is a gateway drug to **sobriety**. That said, *some people may become psychologically dependent on marijuana*, and **this does not mean** that it's a total cure for substance abuse problems; however, from a harm-reduction standpoint, it can be very helpful.

20. Cannabis can stimulate creativity, and improve activity in the brain.

Cannabis usage has actually been shown to have some positive mental effects, particularly in terms of ***stimulating and increasing creativity***. Although people find that short-term memories tend to function worse when high, people improve their function at tests requiring them to come up with new ideas. One study tested participants on their ability to come up with different words related to a concept, and found that cannabis-using people came up with a greater array of related concepts.

Cannabis seems to make the brain better at detecting remote associations that lead to radically new ideas.

Other researchers have found that some people improve their verbal fluency, and their ability to come up with different words, while using cannabis. This may help overcome those disturbing "senior moments." This increase in creative ability and improved brain function may come in part of from the release of dopamine in the brain, lessening inhibitions, and also allowing people to be more relaxed, giving the brain the ability to perceive things differently.

21. Migraine headaches

Migraine headaches that have not responded to other treatments often respond to cannabis by significantly easing, shortening the duration, and in most cases completely relieving them. Replacing more addictive prescription medications with medical cannabis is a far better way to treat any chronic or recurring pain.

Many other uses for medical cannabis

The preceding listing is just a partial inventory of the medical conditions and situations helped by medical cannabis. In the chapter on the states that allow medical marijuana and the conditions for which it can legally be used in those states, you will see a far greater and amazing listing of its uses.

Please note that in any case where you want to try a new treatment approach to any symptom, affliction, or disease, always discuss it with your medical advisor.

Chapter 3.

History of Cannabis as a Medicine

Cannabis is purported by some to have been used as a medicine for perhaps as long as 10,000 years. For sure, 5,000 years ago in China, Emperor Shen Nung prescribed cannabis for **beriberi**, **malaria**, **rheumatism**, **constipation**, **menstrual cramps**, and **absent-mindedness**, among other illnesses. In ancient India, perhaps even earlier, cannabis was used **to lower fevers** and **relieve dysentery**, while in ancient Rome the physician Pedacius Dioscorides prescribed cannabis to treat pain of ***ear ache*** and ***diminished sexual desire***.

Over the following centuries, the use of cannabis as medication had been well accepted, even for the use ***in treatment of tumors***, and a constantly lengthening list of ailments. Its medicinal use spread to Europe and throughout that continent. Eventually, it reached Spain and from there spread to the Caribbean islands, moved on to the South American continent, then up into Mexico. From there, it reached the United States in the early 1800s.

In 1854, the United States Dispensary said about cannabis and its uses:

*"The extract of hemp acts as a decided **aphrodisiac**, **increases the appetite**, and **occasionally induces the cataleptic state**. In morbid states, it has been found **to produce sleep**, **to allay spasm**, **to compose nervous inquietude**, and **to relieve pain**. In these respects it resembles opium in its operation; but it differs from that narcotic in not diminishing the appetite, checking the secretions, or constipating the bowels. It is much less certain in its effects, but may sometimes be preferably employed, when its nauseating or constipating effects contraindicate opium. The complaints to which it has been specially recommended are neuralgia, gout, tetanus, hydrophobia, epidemic cholera,*

convulsions, chorea, hysteria, mental depression, insanity, and uterine hemorrhage". Prof. Alexander Christison of Edinburgh has found it *"***to have the property of hastening**, and **increasing the contractions of the uterus in delivery**. It acts very quickly, and without anesthetic effect. It appears, however, to exert this influence only in a certain proportion of cases."*

***

Cannabis's medical uses were expanded, and it was available in most pharmacies up until 1937. At that time and through 1938, marijuana was made illegal in the United States by act of Congress, in spite of and over the objection of the American Medical Association, which felt its medicinal value for numerous ailments far too beneficial.

Dr. W. C. Woodward of the American Medical Association was the only witness to oppose the bill. The legislative activities committee of the AMA wrote to protest the impending legislation:

"*There is positively* **no evidence to indicate the abuse of cannabis as a medical agent,** *or* **to show that its medicinal use is leading to the development of cannabis addiction.** *Cannabis at the present* *time is slightly used for medicinal purposes, but **it would seem worthwhile to maintain its status as a medicinal agent.** There is a possibility that **a restudy of the drug by modern means may show other advantages to be derived from its medicinal use**.*"

However, **against all the medical advice and objection**, the Marijuana Tax Act was approved by congress in 1937 and cannabis preparations were removed from the United States pharmacopoeia in 1941.

Also in 1941, the LaGuardia Committee took an in-depth look at the marijuana situation in New York, and found **the claims it that caused**

crime, violence, insanity, and death were completely unsubstantiated. As regard to medical use, the LaGuardia report said:

"Marijuana has two qualities which suggest it may have useful actions in man. The first is **the typical euphoria-producing action, which might be applicable in the treatment of various types of mental depression;** the second is **the rather unique property which results in stimulation of appetite.**"

It is of further interesting that **the committee did not shrink from commending euphoria itself as having therapeutic potential**, and **it also noted more than 50 years** *ago the greatest 1990's use of cannabis as an appetite stimulant for patients with cancer, AIDS or Hepatitis C.*

The Controlled Substances Act of 1970 placed illicit drugs into one of five schedule categories, and again the decision as to which schedule a drug was put in was **not made by medical experts,** *but by the Justice Department, the then-Attorney General John Mitchell, and the Bureau of Narcotics and Dangerous Drugs, later named the Drug Enforcement Agency, or DEA*. Cannabis was placed in Schedule I, designated for drugs with a high potential for abuse, and of no medical value.

Almost simultaneously, researchers discovered two new medical uses for cannabis. First was **the ability of cannabis to reduce intraocular pressure**, which recommended its use as a treatment for glaucoma. This led to an interesting legal battle. A schoolteacher, Robert Randall, who suffered from glaucoma, was arrested for **using marijuana to keep from going blind**. He fought his case through the court systems, and in 1976 **forced the federal government to provide him with cannabis for this treatment purpose**, thus becoming **the first legal marijuana smoker in the United States since 1937**.

The second discovery was ***the effect marijuana had on the side effects of over 40 kinds of chemotherapy used as treatments for cancer.*** The most toxic and frequent side effect of chemotherapy is violent, uncontrollable nausea and vomiting often lasting for hours. Often conventional antiemetic treatments didn't help. It was discovered that patients who smoked cannabis before chemotherapy, reported to their doctors that the illegal drug helped them enormously in stopping the vomiting, and even made them hungry (appetite loss also being a problem for chemo patients).

This successful use of cannabis in cancer chemotherapy led to the development of an expensive synthetic tetrahydrocannabinol named **Marinol**, and it was rescheduled into Schedule II. However, the cannabis plant and THC extracted from the natural source, remained in Schedule I.

This well-proven antiemetic significance of cannabis also led to its use by many AIDS patients. In the mid 1980's, cannabis became useful both as an appetite stimulant against the AIDS wasting syndrome, and as a remedy against the intense nausea often caused by HIV's takeover of the immune system, as well as the toxicity of AZT therapy.

Consider the risks

Though a rapidly growing number of doctors and patients recognize that cannabis has many legitimate medical and therapeutic uses, the United States government still disagrees. Federal law still recognizes marijuana as a Schedule I drug, classifying it among the most dangerous drugs that have no recognized medical qualities or uses. If you do not live in one of the growing number of states that have made medical marijuana use legal, you take a risk using marijuana for any purpose, medical or recreational. If you are discovered by law-enforcement officers, with marijuana in your possession in any form, the penalty can range from a small fine to a lengthy prison sentence.

However, the use of hemp oil CBD **is legal in all 50 of the United States**, and may offer the same benefits to you as medical marijuana, and at a much lower cost.

Using cannabis may pose some health risks in rare cases, and so you should always discuss its use with your own medical advisor who knows your personal health situation well. There are several possible consequences to consider, especially for patients with high risk factors for certain illnesses, or in situations where coordination or reasoning are important, including:

1. **Impairment of thinking and problem-solving skills, and memory or reduced balance and coordination**. Cannabis **should never be used** within hours of driving, using dangerous tools.

2. **Increased risk of heart attack.** There is some evidence that there might be increased risk of heart attack in patients that have high risk factors for heart disease.

3. **Heightened risk of chronic cough and respiratory infections.**

4. **Potential for hallucinations, especially with high THC varieties.**

5. **Marijuana smoke contains some of the carcinogenic

hydrocarbons found in tobacco smoke. If you have been a chronic smoker, it might be wise for you to use orally ingested cannabis or vaporized cannabis.

Talk to Your Health Care Professional about Using Medical Marijuana or any form of cannabis!

Chapter 4.

Considering Hemp Oil CBD over Marijuana as Medication

Hemp Oil CBD

This high CBD product comes from the ***agricultural or industrial hemp plant.*** Its ratio CBD to THC is virtually 100% CBD to 0% THC, and since the THC has been almost all bred out of it, this product is legal in all 50 states. It is virtually incapable of causing a high or psychoactive response; however its CBD effects are fully active. Hemp oil CBD can be delivered by ***vaporizer***, ***oil drops***,

salves and ointments, or ***pills and edibles***.

Very Old "New Kid on the Block", Hemp Oil CBD

There is a very bright future for this 5,000-year-old botanical wonder. The fact that industrial hemp oil CBD has the ability to interact with numerous organ systems in the human body, combined with its safety and exceptionally low toxicity, could make it the upcoming miracle medication.

Industrial hemp and medical marijuana both come from the ***Cannabis Sativa L.*** plant, but there is a significant difference.

Agricultural or industrial hemp, often referred to as "**hemp stalk**," grows differently than the THC-containing cannabis, and looks more like bamboo than the familiar looking pot plant. The more familiar looking THC-producing marijuana plants grow to an average of five feet in height, and for best production are spaced six-to-eight feet apart. On the other hand, agricultural hemp grows to a height of 10-to-15 feet or taller when ready for harvest, and can be grown three-to-six inches apart. But most important, agricultural or industrial hemp has **virtually no potential to produce high-content THC** when pollinated by members of their own variety. With proper reproduction, the genetics will remain similar with **virtually no levels of THC**. Because of that fact, hemp oil CBD is legal in all 50 United States. Hemp oil CBD does not require physician's prescription or state registration for purchase or use.

Cannabidiol or CBD, also referred to as a "*phytocannabinoid*," is a plant derivative that can affect appetite, metabolism, pain sensation, inflammation, thermoregulation, vision, mood, and memory, among other aspects of health and body function.

Other differences between marijuana and agricultural hemp

Agricultural or industrial hemp and marijuana come from the same genus of plant designated cannabis. The term "*genus*" refers to a family of plants species and not a single species. In other words, this means that there are multiple types of the cannabis plant, all of which are cannabis, but each having noteworthy differences. The genus of cannabis is includes three distinct species of the cannabis plant: *Cannabis sativa*, *Cannabis indica,* and *Cannabis ruderalis*.

Cannabis sativa is the most commonly known strain of cannabis.

It has been cultivated throughout known history numerous uses, which include **the production of seed oil**, **food**, **hemp fiber** used for **clothes**, **paper**, and **rope**, for **medicine**, and **recreation**.

Cannabis ruderalis on the other hand is a species native to Russia and ***is the hardiest of the three***, and ***is able to withstand far harsher conditions*** than Cannabis sativa or Cannabis indica, but it is relatively poor in cannabinoids **having a lower THC content** than either sativa or indica.

Cannabis indica, as its name indicates, was discovered in India and is a cannabis species that ***is shorter and bushier than sativa***.

Some scientists doubt the existence of Cannabis indica as a distinct and separate species of cannabis.

In nature, Cannabis ruderalis characteristically has the lowest levels of THC, while Cannabis sativa has a higher level of THC than CBD, and Cannabis indica has a higher level of CBD than THC. That's in nature, however, since man has been cultivating cannabis, especially Cannabis sativa, for thousands of years, the effects of man-made pollination selections have led to several different types of cannabis within the same species. These artificial pollinations have been designer selections aimed at goals depending on the purpose the cannabis was cultivated for.

Artificial selection

Humans have cultivated cannabis since antiquity, and for a variety of purposes. Through artificial selection, different species of cannabis have different properties; some have been used for medicinal purposes, others as food, and others to create clothes, ropes, and other industrial substances.

Industrial hemp has been produced by strains of Cannabis sativa that have been cultivated to produce very minimal levels of THC, and have been artificially selected and bred to grow taller and sturdier. This has enabled the plant to be used successfully in the production of hemp oil, wax, resin, hemp seed food, animal feed, fuel, cloth, rope, paper, and much more. Industrial hemp is exclusively bred from Cannabis sativa.

Medical marijuana is produced mainly from variants of Cannabis sativa, which have been selectively bred to maximize their varying concentration in cannabinoids. Cannabis ruderalis is almost exclusively grown for medicinal purposes, since it naturally has very small quantities of THC. The major difference then between industrial hemp and medical marijuana is that industrial hemp is exclusively made from Cannabis sativa that was specifically bred to produce the lowest concentrations of THC possible. Industrial hemp always has trace amounts of THC and naturally occurring high amounts of CBD having the highest CBD/THC ratio of all cannabis strains. This means that industrial hemp's chemical profile makes it incapable of inducing intoxicating effects and getting you "high" from ingesting it, thus making it legal in all 50 United States.

Industrial Hemp Dietary Supplements

Industrial hemp is naturally rich in CBD and has only trace amounts of THC. Many patients are turning to industrial hemp products as alternatives to medical marijuana. Since medical marijuana is not legal in all the states in the US or in many countries worldwide, products made from industrial hemp can be a safe and legal alternative. Patients can get most of the same beneficial effects of medical marijuana from industrial hemp products, and without getting the high.

Industrial hemp products are safe, are made according to federal standards, and are produced in FDA-registered facilities within the US.

The Many Medical Benefits of CBD

Research is still scratching the surface, but cannabidiol is proving to be immensely beneficial for the treatment of many different ailments and disorders, matching most if not all treated by medical marijuana. ***Its anticonvulsant benefits for children and adults*** are getting most of the headlines about CBD oil being ***available to children suffering from epilepsy.*** CBD oil can also ***treat inflammation***, ***pain***, ***anxiety***, ***many neurodegenerative*** *disorders*, *PTSD*, *sleep disorders*, *arthritis*, *fibromyalgia* and *nightmares*, to name just a few. It has even been *linked to the treatment of cancer*, easing its pain, *nausea of chemotherapy*, and *curbing the loss of appetite*. Some studies suggest that CBD *retards the growth of cancer* and *may even* **kill** *cancer cells.*

Hemp CBD is available as **oil** and as a **pill**. CBD oil used *to treat intractable epilepsy*, for example, is administered a few drops at a time with the help of a dropper. **No smoking need be involved**; however, it can be delivered *as a vapor* using a small vaporizer a little larger than a cigarette holder.

CBD from Medical Marijuana Is Still Illegal In Many States

Though CBD or cannabidiol *obtained from industrial hemp* **is legal** and considered a dietary supplement, CBD *obtained from marijuana* **is not**. This is, as mentioned before, because CBD from hemp contains **virtually no THC** while that obtained from medical marijuana may contain large concentrations of THC. In states where it is legal, CBD from medical marijuana is dispensed only to those who are able to get a doctor's prescription.

Chapter 5.
Hemp and Marijuana Delivery Methods

Pure hemp cannabidiol oil can be consumed directly as a nutritional supplement. Over the years, great advances in CBD hemp oil product development have led to what are now dozens of different types of CBD hemp oil products, including **capsules**, **drops**, and **even chewing gum**. Concentrated CBD hemp oil can also be infused into **skin and body care products** and used topically.

Our understanding of CBD cannabis oil has expanded, and we're more aware today than ever of the cannabinoids potential. Studies on CBD's natural health benefits are extensive, and groundbreaking research is being done regularly. We suggest you **review the wide body of scientific research on CBD** to get a better understanding of the cannabinoid's health value.

Hemp CBD and Marijuana Delivery Methods

When it comes to cannabis consumption, the delivery method is perhaps the next most important consideration. If you find yourself within this category but aspire to become a comprehensive cannabis aficionado, let this be your checklist. Gaining maximum benefits of medical cannabis largely depends on how it's consumed. Each method of consumption provides unique effects.

The three basic delivery methods are **inhalation**, **oral**, and **topical**. Under these three umbrella delivery methods are various sub-techniques, each appropriate for different purposes.

Inhalation delivery methods

When cannabis is inhaled, **the smoke or vapors enter the lungs to be absorbed into the bloodstream**. The two established types of inhalation methods are **smoking** and **vaporization**.

Smoking method

This is the most common method of inhalation associated with cannabis. Health professionals are in general agreement that ***smoke-free methods pose less health risk*** and ***are medically preferred***.

There are a wide assortment of devices at the smoker's preference, including **hand pipes**, **water pipes**, **rolling papers**, **hookahs**, and **homemade devices**.

Hand Pipes

These are probably the most common smoking devices used today and are favored for their convenience. They are small, easily manageable, simple-to-carry, and use. They function by carrying the smoke created from burning cannabis in their bowls, which is then inhaled by the consumer. Their function is not unlike a tobacco smoker's pipe, though they come in a multitude of designs, very different from tobacco pipes.

Water Pipes

Like hand pipes, water pipes come in a large variety of styles and designs, but they are increased in complexity by incorporating water as a filter. The health benefits associated with the addition of water are questionable. Water tends to cool the smoke, but it is debatable if it is really an effective filter for harmful components.

Rolling Papers

Rolling papers are generally used to smoke joints, which are cannabis rolled in a thin paper. Blunts are cannabis rolled in cigar paper actually made from tobacco leaf and thus contain nicotine. Blunt smokers prefer the flavor, smell, and combined effects of the nicotine and cannabis. The added medical risks linked to nicotine and other tobacco carcinogens discourage most health-conscious cannabis consumers.

Hookahs

This is one of the least used methods of smoking cannabis. Cannabis is seldom smoked alone in a hookah because the plant burns faster than it can be inhaled, producing an acrid taste, and too great a wasting of the product, as large quantities of marijuana are needed to yield the same results as other smoking methods. To resolve this economic problem, cannabis is often sandwiched between tobacco, which introduces the same health concerns associated with blunts.

Homemade One-Time Use Devices

This includes all cannabis-smoking devices that are homemade, or adapted to deliver cannabis smoke to the user. The method allows for the greatest creativity, and there is probably no limit to inventions and gadgets used, but the most common homemade device is some form of pipe due to its simplicity.

Vaporization

Since hemp oil CBD is not used in leaf or seed form, the aforementioned methods of smoking do not apply to hemp oil CBD users.

Vaporization is **the logical choice for health-conscious cannabis consumers**, be they marijuana or hemp users. A vaporizer heats cannabis to a temperature that is high enough to extract the THC, CBD, and other cannabinoids, but is kept too low to burn the marijuana, keeping the potentially harmful toxins that are released in smoke from combustion. In other words, vaporization eliminates the health risks associated with smoking. A side benefit comes with a significant reduction in the cannabis-burning odor. There are an expanding variety of vaporizer types as the technology improves. Many vaporizers take cannabis concentrates, which come in a variety of forms including oil and wax.

Oral Delivery Methods

Oral delivery includes all products that are administered through the mouth, which include ***tinctures***, ***ingestible oils***, and ***cannabis-infused foods and drinks***. Tinctures are essentially a topical application that is administered through the mouth, but they are immediately absorbed into the bloodstream through the oral mucosal membranes, unlike edibles or drinks, which are absorbed in the stomach.

Tinctures

Tinctures are liquid cannabis extracts used by consumers seeking both dosage control and a fast-acting effect, without the health risks associated with smoking. Most commonly, alcohol of proof greater than 80 is used as the solvent, but other fat-soluble liquids can be used as well, such as vinegar or glycerol. Generally, just three or four drops of the tincture are placed under the tongue, where it is directly absorbed into the body instead of being swallowed and digested. Ingested, tinctures are instantly absorbed in an empty stomach but still require time to be processed through the liver, thus reducing dosage control.

Ingestible Oils

Ingestible oils are an in-between method to edibles and tinctures in that **they are swallowed and digested like an infused product, but often have the consistency of oil.** These oils can either be eaten or put in easily swallowed capsules.

Edibles

Edibles can be defined as **any food that contains cannabis.** These products have a considerably longer onset and tend to cause longer effects.

Infused food and drinks can be made a variety of ways, but most often, edibles are **infused using an** *ingredient high in fat* (such as butter or olive oil) *that enable extraction of the plant's therapeutic properties*. Adding tinctures to foods is another option for dosage control and simplicity. Keep in mind that eaten cannabis is absorbed slowly through the stomach, especially after eating other food. People used to smoking cannabis may feel that they haven't had enough orally ingested cannabis after not feeling its effect in a few minutes, and so they take more of the edible, which can lead to overdosing, which can in turn cause a serious high, and even hallucinations if THC is an ingredient.

Topical Delivery Methods

Topical cannabis administration utilizes a thick oil extract that has been decarboxylated to activate cannabinoids. Once the cannabinoids are activated, they can be absorbed ***through your skin***.

The topical effects of cannabis differ from other medicating methods in that they do not provide the cerebral stimulation that users describe as being high. Topicals are appropriate ***for consumers needing a clear head and localized relief, such as muscle aches or joint soreness***.

Chapter 6.

Who Should Not Use Hemp Oil CBD or Marijuana?

Hemp oil CBD or medicinal marijuana therapy isn't for everyone, and specifically not for you if you have some condition that could get worse with the use of cannabis, or in cases where the risks might outweigh the benefits. That's true for any type of medical treatment, conventional medical methods included.

Also patients who have pre-existing psychiatric disorders like *schizophrenia*, or who have a *strong family history of mental illness*, or who **might have bad reactions to cannabis**. That is not to say they shouldn't use medical cannabis, but their ***private physician or mental health counselor should very carefully monitor them***.

Medical cannabis therapy should be absolutely contraindicated for ***patients who have a severe allergy to the pollen in cannabis or to any of the compounds in cannabis***. Also, if medical marijuana ***interferes with some essential other type of therapy that the patient needs*** it should be contraindicated, or overall therapy should be reviewed with the prescribing physician or physicians. In some states, transplant candidates awaiting organ transplants *may be disqualified if there is marijuana in their system*.

Keep in mind that *there remains a conflict here between federal and the state law when it comes to the use of marijuana as a medicine*. Presently, it is the administration's policy to not interfere with state laws, but if a more conservative administration is elected in the future that may change. If you are made anxious by this risk, though it is not presently great, then use of medical marijuana is probably not right for you at this time. However, if you and your medical advisors feel that the benefits to you do indeed outweigh these risks, therapy might be right for you. This is where hemp oil CBD is of great advantage since it is legal in all 50 of the United States of America!

Who Should Definitely Avoid Cannabis Use?

Healthy Teens

While cannabis consumption is far safer than many things teens will experiment with, there is some evidence that teens who consume cannabis before the age of 16 are susceptible to permanent changes in the brain. Some researchers suggest that heavy use of marijuana before the age of 25 might lead to permanent brain changes or personality changes. More research in this area is needed. However, promising areas for the treatment children and teens with cannabis include **treatment of epilepsy**, **cancer**, **autism**, and other select diseases where cannabis can provide incredible symptomatic relief, and in some cases can markedly alter the disease process. Cannabinoids should also be used cautiously, especially in teens, if there is a family history of psychosis, or if any user is at a high risk of developing psychosis.

Anyone Wishing To Become Pregnant

There is actually little scientific evidence on this subject; however, it is probably wise to err on the side of caution for anyone who wants to conceive. Preliminary research raises the concern that due to the high anti-angiogenic effect of cannabis, which prevents growth of new blood vessels, it is thought that cannabis use could prevent the egg's adhesion to the uterine wall and lead to a miscarriage.

Elderly people

Seniors should keep in mind that *cannabis may cause dizziness*, or *could affect their balance*. For this reason, they should take all necessary precautions to ensure their safety when using cannabis.

Chapter 7.

Why Marijuana was Made Illegal in the United States

To understand the marijuana laws in the United States today, we have to go back to the early 1900's, shortly following the Mexican Revolution, which caused an influx of immigration from Mexico into southern states like Texas and Louisiana. Of course, these new immigrants brought with them their native language, culture, and customs, but also the use of marijuana as a medicine and relaxant.

At the time, Americans were quite familiar with cannabis ***as a medication***, since it was present in almost all tinctures and medicines at the time; but the word ***marijuana*** was foreign to them. And to many Americans, these new immigrants created fear and bigotry.

Following the fear and bigotry, the media began to play on the fears that the public had about these new citizens, spreading false claims about these "*troublesome and dangerous Mexicans with their dodgy native behaviors*", including the use of marijuana. What the majority of the rest of the nation didn't know was that **this** marijuana was the same they had in their medicine cabinets.

Actually, the United States Census of 1850 counted **8,327 hemp plantations** that were growing cannabis hemp for ***cloth***, ***canvas***, and even **the cordage used for baling cotton**.

Thus, the demonization of the cannabis plant was a natural expansion of the demonization of the Mexican immigrants. In their effort to control these new immigrants, El Paso, Texas did what San Francisco, California did to control Chinese immigrants, which was to outlawed opium decades earlier. The idea was to have an excuse to search, detain and deport

Mexican immigrants, and like opium to control the Chinese, that excuse was marijuana.

Among the first state laws outlawing marijuana may have been influenced, not only by Mexicans using cannabis, but also because of Mormons using it. Some Mormons who traveled to Mexico in 1910 came back to Salt Lake City with marijuana. The church's reaction to this may have contributed to that state's marijuana laws.

Other states quickly followed suit with marijuana prohibition laws, including Wyoming (1915), Texas (1919), Iowa (1923), Nevada (1923), Oregon (1923), Washington (1923), Arkansas (1923), and

Nebraska (1927). From bigotry and fear, these laws tended to be specifically targeted against the Mexican-American population.

In the eastern states, the *"marijuana problem"* was attributed to the Latin Americans and Black jazz musicians. Marijuana and jazz musicians who used it freely, traveled from New Orleans via Kansas City to Chicago, and then on to Harlem, where marijuana seemed to become a key part of the popular music scene. And again, racism became a major part of the indictment against marijuana. Newspaper editorial columns proclaimed, *"Marijuana influences Negroes to look at white people in the eye, step on white men's shadows, and look at a white woman twice."*

An additional fear-tactic, which was spread through the media, was that Mexicans, Blacks, and other foreigners were introducing white children to marijuana, and marijuana was linking them to violent behavior.

The Federal Approaches to Drug Prohibition

In 1930, a new division in the Treasury Department was established; it was named the Federal Bureau of Narcotics, and Harry J. Anslinger was named its director. This marked the beginning of the federal all-out war against marijuana.

Harry J. Anslinger

Anslinger was an extremely ambitious man, and recognized the Bureau of Narcotics as his career opportunity.

He saw his new government agency as his chance to define both the problem and the solution. He came to realize that opiates and cocaine weren't problems enough to build him and his agency's importance, so he hit on marijuana to **make it illegal at the federal level**.

Anslinger immediately turned to the effective themes of **racism and**

violence to draw national attention to the marijuana problem he needed to create. He promoted wild tales of "ax murderers on marijuana", and sex, and Mexicans, and Negroes, and foreigners, and violence. Among the quotes he spread that have been attributed to Anslinger and his Gore Files:

"There are 100,000 total marijuana smokers in the US, and most are Negroes, Hispanics, Filipinos, and entertainers. Their Satanic music, jazz and swing, result from marijuana use. This marijuana causes white women to seek sexual relations with Negroes, entertainers, and many others. The primary reason to outlaw marijuana is its effect on the degenerate races.

"Marijuana is an addictive drug which produces in its user's insanity, criminality, and death. Reefer makes darkies think they're as good as white men.

"Marijuana leads to pacifism and communist brainwashing. You smoke a joint, and you're likely to kill your brother. Marijuana is the most violence-causing drug in the history of mankind."

And he used his favorite version of the definition of the word "***assassin***":

"In the year 1090, there was founded in Persia the religious and military order of **the Assassins**, whose history is one of cruelty, barbarity, and murder, and for good reason: the members were confirmed users of hashish, or marijuana, and it is from the Arabs' 'hashashin' that we have the English word 'assassin.'"

Self-Serving Yellow Journalism

Harry Anslinger got some additional and timely help from William Randolph Hearst, who owned a chain of newspapers. And Hearst had lots of personal reasons to help Anslinger.

First, and probably most important, he was heavily invested in the timber industry to support his newspaper chain, and **didn't want to see the development of hemp paper as competition**. Secondly, **he had lost 800,000 acres of timberland to Poncho Villa**, so he hated Mexicans. And then, **telling lurid lies about immigrant Mexicans and the** "devil marijuana weed drug causing violence" **sold newspapers**, which made him wealthier.

This campaign of bigotry and invented violence became the major force in passing the Marijuana Tax Act of 1937, which effectively banned its possession, use, and sales.

Years later, this Act was **ruled unconstitutional**, so it was replaced with the Controlled Substances Act in the 1970's, which established the Schedules for classifying substances according to their danger and potential for addiction. Cannabis was then placed in the most restrictive category, Schedule I.

Although the Schafer Commission *declared that marijuana should not be in Schedule I*, and even *declined its designation as an illicit substance*, President Nixon discounted the report of the commission, and its recommendations, and so marijuana remained, and still remains a Schedule I substance.

The use of hemp oil CBD has never been against the laws of any of the United States; however, **the growing of hemp in the United States has been illegal or under strict state and federal control.**

Chapter 8.

Is Cannabis a Gateway Drug, or Addictive?

Although there are some correlations between marijuana and other addictive drugs, there is no conclusive evidence that one actually causes the other.

The gateway theory refers to the idea that marijuana, in this case, leads its users to eventually abuse other addictive drugs. Though studies of large populations have indeed found that some of those who smoke marijuana are more likely to use other drugs, these studies show a correlation **but not**

causation. The fallacy is, just because marijuana smokers might be more likely to later use cocaine, or some other drug, **does not imply that using marijuana causes one to use these other drugs**.

A 1999 report from the Institute of Medicine, a branch of the National Academy of Sciences, stated clearly, *"In the sense that marijuana use typically precedes rather than follows initiation into the use of other illicit drugs, it is indeed a gateway drug. However, it does not appear to be a gateway drug to the extent that it is the cause or even that it is the most significant predictor of serious drug abuse; that is, care must be taken not to attribute cause to association."*

The scientific community shares no consensus on the issue of marijuana being a gateway drug, and there is little evidence on the underlying cause and effect.

Social and cultural concerns

The cultural and social concerns pointing to a gateway theory point to the possibility that simply by being around marijuana, and the people who use it, one might be more likely to end up trying other drugs as well. There is also the suggestion that an individual who uses marijuana may simply be a person more likely to engage in risk-taking behavior, and will seek out and experiment with other drugs.

This would suggest there is no causal link from marijuana to other drugs, but rather a social link to people who make it possible to be introduced to other more difficult-to-obtain substances.

An argument for legalizing marijuana is that legal cannabis providers have too much at risk to their licensing to risk selling other illegal drugs, while the street corner illegal provider will try to push the marijuana smoker into more costly, lucrative and addicting drugs. In other words, marijuana's illegal status may contribute to its gateway effects by simply introducing smokers to other illegal drugs, which means a marijuana user would be more likely to have access to other illegal drugs through social interactions, and the act of actually buying the drugs illegally.

A Drug and Alcohol Dependence study found that **marijuana use was far less associated with other illicit drug use in the Netherlands**, where marijuana can legally be purchased in so-called coffee shops, than in other countries including the United States.

More than likely Cannabis is a gateway drug to sobriety!

The fact is that most studies indicate there is **no firm ground to stand on when making claims of marijuana's gateway effect**. In fact, since medical marijuana is being used successfully to help addicts to get off of alcohol and other addictive illegal and prescription drugs, one might say it is a gateway drug to sobriety.

Look for other books in this Hemp Oil CBD series as they are published:

1. Hemp Oil CBD (Legal in all 50 United States) vs. Medical Marijuana

2. **Sleep Deprivation Management with Hemp Oil CBD**

3. **Cancer Treatment with Hemp Oil CBD**

4. **Pain Management with Hemp Oil CBD**

5. **Inflammation Management with Hemp Oil CBD**

6. **PTSD Treatment with Hemp Oil CBD**

7. **Alzheimer's And Parkinson's Management and Other Neurological Diseases with Hemp Oil CBD**

About the Author

Othniel Seiden, MD has practiced medicine for over 45 years; first in General Practice, and then as an Emergency Physician. He, in fact, is a Charter Member of The American College of Emergency Physicians, started when Emergency Medicine first became a specialty. During his years as a physician; he also had over 30 books published: five historical novels and over 25 non-fiction publications. Also, in 1981, Dr. Seiden founded Doctors To The World, a 501(C)(3) charitable organization still active today bringing medical help into disadvantaged areas all over the world.

Dr. Seiden lectures on the numerous subjects of his publications now numbering over 70 published books. All of his books can be seen on Amazon.com and by Googling him.

Hemp Oil CBD (Legal in all 50 United States) vs. Medical Marijuana©

is also available for purchase at PachydermPublishing.com

and in Kindle form at Amazon.com

www.ingramcontent.com/pod-product-compliance
Lightning Source LLC
Chambersburg PA
CBHW070301230526
45470CB00002B/665